ESSENTIAL BLOOD PRESSURE SOLUTION

A Comprehensive Approach To
Understanding, Managing, And
Preventing, Your Blood Pressure Naturally
Without Medication

By
Kathy Dang

Table Of Contents

Introduction

The saying that high blood pressure is the ultimate silent killer is one that we have all heard. Not only does it impact one in three individuals in your vicinity, but it also plays a role in heart disease, diabetes, coronary heart disease, kidney failure, and—above all—destroys your only opportunity to lead a typical, healthy life. Learn as much as you can about high blood pressure, its permanent repercussions, and how to stop it before it starts. Start examining yourself; the routines you've developed and their effects on your arterial walls. Recognize the toll your lifestyle and dietary choices are taking on your heart and the rest of your body, and make the necessary changes to move toward a healthier and happier life.

Because blood pressure drugs target symptoms rather than the underlying cause, they are typically highly dangerous and unable to permanently control blood pressure. In addition, a lot of these blood pressure drugs have long-lasting adverse effects that might make living less enjoyable. The secret is to use a variety of natural remedies that work in concert to lower high blood pressure.

This book will expose the truth about salt, which is a substance that can be found in all of your food items, including candies, frozen meals, and potato chips. Recognize that no two sodium particles are the same. Between table salt and "sea salt," there is a huge difference that could inspire you to try new, colorful ways to season your food. Additionally, you'll start to learn how to manage your salting experiences to balance your cells and detoxify your body. This equilibrium can make you feel better and more energized while also lowering blood pressure.

You'll discover which herbs and oils will assist in naturally lowering your blood pressure, as well as appropriate lifestyle changes. Additionally, you will discover how to design a heart-healthy lifestyle that emphasizes physical activity, a wholesome diet, wise decision-making, and improved long-term health. Additionally, this book contains twenty delectable heart-healthy recipes that you can make to enhance your life with superfoods that naturally lower your blood pressure—without the need for potent pharmaceuticals. Learn how to make low-sodium meals, appetizers, and desserts.

You can regulate your blood pressure. You can bring it down, make it normal, and guarantee yourself better health in the future. Your high blood pressure does not mean the end of your life. But your former existence—enriched with excessive amounts of booze, table salt, and culinary selections—is no longer here. Find the courage to proceed!

CHAPTER 1:

BLOOD PRESSURE: NUMBERS, FACTS, AND FIGURES

Millions of individuals worldwide suffer from the extremely prevalent ailment known as high blood pressure. Remarkably, just around half of adult Americans with high blood pressure today have their condition under control. Approximately one in three adults in America suffer from high blood pressure. In short, high blood pressure is a powerful push of blood against the walls of your arteries, which can cause heart failure, stroke, coronary heart disease, renal failure, and other issues. Primarily, high blood pressure typically exhibits no symptoms, hence many sufferers are not aware of their condition.

How Is Blood Pressure Calculated?

Blood pressure is essentially a battle between the volume of blood the heart pumps through the body and the amount of resistance the arteries erect to that volume of blood. The body's total blood pressure soars as a result of the arteries being extremely constricted because the body finds it difficult to pump blood through them. Just consider this: if water were poured into a thick drain, the water would flow through with little resistance. That being said, water would find it difficult to pass through a thin tube if it were forced through. The strain would increase.

Blood Pressure By The Numbers

Systolic and diastolic blood pressure measurements are used to calculate the scientific measurement of blood pressure. Systolic blood pressure is what the body experiences during a heartbeat. The blood pressure that the body experiences during its resting state between pumps is known as diastolic. Typically, the systolic and diastolic numbers are written above each other, resulting in the following:

75/115 mmHg. The term "millimeters of mercury" (mmHG) should be noted.

Systolic and diastolic blood pressure readings less than or equal to 120 mm Hg and 80 mm Hg, respectively, are indicative of optimum blood pressure.

	Systolic		Diastolic	
Optimal	<120	&	<80	
Normal	<130	&	<85	
Prehyperten sion	130-139	or	85-89	
Stage 1	140-159	or	90-99	
Stage 2	160-179	or	100-109	

The risk of high blood pressure varies throughout phases. Prehypertension, for instance, is present in those with systolic values between 130 and 139 OR diastolic values between 85 and 89. As a result, their chance of getting high blood pressure and hypertension is significantly increased.

Additionally, a person is classified as having stage 1 high blood pressure if their diastolic blood pressure is between 90 and 99 and their systolic blood pressure is between 140 and 159.

People with stage 2 high blood pressure have systolic blood pressure values greater than 160 OR diastolic blood pressure values greater than 100. Stage 2 is considerably riskier and more challenging to manage than stage 1.

But keep in mind that blood pressure fluctuates constantly. For example, blood pressure rises when you wake up from sleep and falls when you wake up. Additionally, blood pressure increases in tense, agitated, or active states. A persistently high number increases the likelihood of major health issues. If a person's blood pressure is in the prehypertensive range, they need to act quickly to lower it to prevent further issues related to high blood pressure.

Congratulations if you have ever experienced high blood pressure and you have taken the necessary actions to lower it. It's crucial to keep in mind, though, that those who have already experienced high blood pressure are always affected by the illness. Continuous adherence to treatment strategies is necessary to prevent high blood pressure.

Why Should You Care About High Blood Pressure?

Recall that around 348,000 American deaths in 2009 were attributable to excessive blood pressure. This indicates that 1,000 individuals were wiped by excessive blood pressure every single day of that year.

Furthermore, high blood pressure is linked to heart attacks in seven out of ten cases of first-time heart attack victims; it is also linked to strokes in eight out of ten cases; and it is present in seven out of ten cases of chronic heart failure patients. They wouldn't have had these excruciating medical ailments if they had changed their way of life, made better dietary

and exercise choices, and kept their blood pressure
in check.

CHAPTER 2:

THE QUIET KILLER: SEARCHING FOR SIGNS AND SYMPTOMS OF HIGH BLOOD PRESSURE

Keep in mind that there are no obvious symptoms or indicators of high blood pressure. Sometimes, folks get headaches all the time. These headaches, though, might indicate other medical conditions. Of course, the last thing that comes to mind when someone has a headache is to check their blood pressure.

As a result, people may have high blood pressure for a long time without realizing they have the condition. Increased blood pressure damages the heart, kidneys, blood vessels, and other organs, resulting in more severe health problems. Most people, in general, don't become aware of their high blood pressure until they visit their doctor to address one of these later conditions.

Therefore, it's critical to always be aware of your blood pressure readings. As you age and become more vulnerable to high blood pressure, you should work with a physician, a team of healthcare providers, and a suitable lifestyle plan to maintain your normal blood pressure readings.

Consult Your Doctor

People should discuss blood pressure with their doctor after turning eighteen and request a reading every two years. It is important to take a blood pressure reading from each arm to identify any variations. Keep in mind that higher blood pressure is warranted by a history of readings more frequently. Additionally, blood pressure checks will occasionally be offered by other community organizations or at health resource fairs. It is imperative to regularly check your levels, even if you don't see your doctor very often. It should be noted that individuals should refrain from smoking or consuming coffee one hour before the test to maintain normal blood pressure levels. Furthermore, because moving about might cause blood pressure to rise, individuals should sit still for at least five minutes before the test.

Blood Pressure Effects Over Time

Recognize the following harm that, if untreated, high blood pressure can cause over time:

1. Aneurysms

Aneurysms in blood arteries can develop as a result of high blood pressure. A large bubble-shaped bulging in the arterial wall is called an aneurysm. These aneurysms typically occur in the principal arteries that supply blood to the brain, the intestines, the legs, and the spleen, as well as the blood vessel that distributes blood throughout the body from the heart.

2. Big, Weak Heart

The heart is significantly more prone to failing when it grows weak and enlarged. The body goes into oxygen deprivation mode when heart failure prevents the heart from pumping enough blood to the rest of the body.

3. Narrow Kidney Blood Vessels

The body is more likely to experience renal failure when the blood arteries in the kidneys narrow.

4. Burst Eye Blood Vessels

There is a serious chance of blindness or vision changes when the blood vessels in the eyes burst.

5. Increased Risk of Stroke, Heart Attack, and Leg Amputation

Reduced blood flow can result from high blood pressure narrowing the arteries throughout the body. The body is more vulnerable to heart attacks, strokes, and amputations of the legs when there is insufficient blood flow.

6. Loss of Understanding and Memory

Uncontrolled hypertension causes a person's memory and comprehension to start to decline.

CHAPTER 3:

AM I AT RISK? UNDERSTANDING HIGH BLOOD PRESSURE TARGETS

Over the world, millions of people suffer from high blood pressure. Currently, one in three adult Americans suffers from this illness and battles daily to improve their health.

Understanding Who Is At Risk For High Blood Pressure

1. Some Races or Ethnicities Are More Affected by High Blood Pressure Than Others

Remember that anyone, regardless of color, can have high blood pressure. However, compared to most Hispanic or Caucasian individuals, African-American adults are significantly more likely to suffer from excessive blood pressure. It is clear from examining the numbers that:

A: A higher incidence of high blood pressure is seen in adult African Americans early in life.

B: Adult African Americans have higher levels of severe high blood pressure.

C: Adult African Americans have a lower ability to manage their hypertension with drugs and other therapies.

D: Adult African Americans are more likely to die from high blood pressure. These fatalities include kidney failure, diabetes, coronary heart disease, and stroke.

Keep in mind that various Hispanic American adults are also at varying risk of hypertension. Adults of Puerto Rican descent, for instance, are more likely than members of other Hispanic populations to die from high blood pressure. All Caucasians have a higher risk of dying from high blood pressure than Cuban Americans.

2. High blood pressure risks increase with age

Research indicates that over 65 percent of Americans who are older than sixty experience excessive blood pressure. These elderly people typically experience isolated systolic hypertension, a particular type of high blood pressure that arises when the systolic blood pressure, or the top number in the reading, is very high.

Keep in mind that at this later age, high blood pressure is not always the result. Preventive measures are crucial in mitigating dangers from previous years.

3. Gender Influences High Blood Pressure Numbers

There is no difference in the likelihood of developing high blood pressure in men and women over time. However, the duration of the affliction varies according to their gender. It should be noted that women are far more likely than males to experience high blood pressure after the age of sixty-five, while men are much less likely to experience it in this age range.

4: The Number on the Scale Affects High Blood Pressure Risks

Obese or overweight people are considerably more likely to get high blood pressure problems. A person who is overweight or obese has a weight that is higher than normal for their skeletal build and bone structure.

5. Lifestyle Irresponsibilities Increase the Risk of High Blood Pressure

Individuals who lead unsuitable lifestyles are more likely to develop hypertension. For instance, if they

A. Smoke Cigarette

Smoking causes a rapid rise in blood pressure. The chemicals in tobacco can eventually cause damage to the lining of the arteries, narrowing them and raising blood pressure.

B. Consume excessive amounts of liquor, wine, or beer

High blood pressure may eventually result from men consuming more than two alcoholic beverages daily and women consuming more than one.

C. Have a potassium deficiency in their diet

The body's cells can maintain a balanced sodium level thanks to potassium. Pumping blood maintains too many sodium particles in the absence of potassium.

D. Consume too much salt and sodium

The body is forced to hold onto liquids by salt. The blood pressure is raised by this fluid retention.

E. Do not Exercise

Frequent exercisers have slower heart rates. The heart has to work harder to beat and pump blood via the arteries if there is no activity. This increases the force and raises blood pressure.

F. Don't get enough vitamin D

It has been demonstrated that vitamin D modifies a kidney enzyme that helps maintain normal blood pressure.

G. Have a high level of stress

Higher levels of stress can be automatically attributed to continuous stress. Blood pressure spikes as a result, which over time may turn chronic. Instead of drinking alcohol, smoking cigarettes, or overindulging in unhealthy foods, find alternate ways to decompress and unwind. This way of living choices may cause blood pressure to rise even higher.

Understanding At-Risk Youth

Even though older people are typically affected by high blood pressure, it's crucial to remember that adolescents and teenagers nowadays are more likely to have prehypertension as well as high blood pressure. This is because obesity rates among children and teenagers have risen sharply in recent years as a result of poor eating habits, inactivity, and other lifestyle factors.

Keep in mind that compared to Caucasian youngsters, children and teenagers of Mexican and African American descent are considerably more likely to have high blood pressure. Don't forget to get high blood pressure screenings for kids and teenagers.

Additional Causes of High Blood Pressure

Many medical conditions, including thyroid illness, chronic renal disease, and sleep apnea, can be associated with high blood pressure. Additionally, several cold remedies and asthma medications might raise blood pressure.

Women need to know that certain birth control medications, hormone therapy, and pregnancy might raise blood pressure levels. Women typically see an increase in both their diastolic and systolic blood pressure readings when they start taking birth control. Before taking birth control tablets, women who are at risk for high blood pressure should consult their doctor.

CHAPTER 4:

THE LINK BETWEEN BLOOD PRESSURE, DIABETES, AND CORONARY HEART PROBLEMS

Understanding Coronary Heart Disease

The most prevalent type of heart disease worldwide is coronary heart disease. In the US, it is the primary cause of mortality for both men and women. Plaque accumulation in the coronary arteries surrounding the heart leads to the development of the disease. Every one of these arteries supplies oxygenated blood to the heart. The plaque may harden or crack during plaque accumulation. A blood clot forms at the plaque's surface when it cracks. This clot has the potential to stop the heart's blood supply, removing oxygenated blood from the body. The coronary artery may become even more narrowed and blocked by this burst plaque.

Recall that while the heart pumps blood throughout the body, blood pressure is the result of the blood's ultimate force against the artery walls. When a person has high blood pressure, their arteries are under too much pressure, which affects the health of other body organs. Thus, elevated blood pressure may have a role in the development of coronary heart disease.

This obstruction leads to heart attacks. The attacks cause the cardiac muscles to become permanently damaged. The heart suffers irreversible damage when a clot, spasm, or narrow wall obstructs the coronary artery, depriving it of oxygen.

People who have high blood pressure are more likely to develop atherosclerosis of coronary artery disease.

Increased pressure against these coronary artery walls is further encouraged by high blood pressure. The arteries have a higher chance of narrowing and encouraging heart attack and failure as they harden following the healing of the damage caused by high blood pressure.

Further obstructing blood flow to other bodily areas like the kidneys and brain are these damaged arteries. Further consequences from this include renal disorders, blindness, and congestive heart failure.

The Connection Between Diabetes and Blood Pressure

Individuals who have diabetes either don't produce enough insulin, have excessive blood sugar levels, or don't react to insulin in the bloodstream well enough. Diabetes, which causes elevated blood sugar levels, impacts more than 300 million individuals globally. Moreover, blood pressure has to be regularly checked since diabetics are far more likely to develop cardiovascular disease.

High blood pressure can exacerbate diabetic consequences such as kidney and eye problems, as well as exacerbate symptoms of the condition. In addition, a large percentage of individuals with diabetes eventually acquire high blood pressure. This is due to the way diabetes affects arteries, increasing their vulnerability to atherosclerosis, or the hardening of the arteries. High blood pressure raises the risk of heart failure, stroke, blood vessel damage, and renal failure. Atherosclerosis can increase this risk. To prevent heart attacks and strokes, people with diabetes should keep an eye on their blood pressure measurements. Their diastolic pressure should not exceed 80, and their systolic pressure should not exceed 140. Diabetes sufferers should be aware that blood pressure readings are just as crucial to preserving good health as blood sugar readings.

CHAPTER 5:

REBUKE MEDICATION: THE SEARCH FOR AT-HOME, NATURAL BLOOD PRESSURE SOLUTIONS

Blood Pressure Medication: Why Is Going Natural Always Better?

To decrease their high blood pressure, many people with high blood pressure seek help from medical professionals. Doesn't it seem evident that this? Ultimately, blood pressure drugs appear to be a quick route to improved health. Medications for high blood pressure include, for example:

1. Beta-blockers

Beta-blockers lessen nerve impulses and slow down your heart rate. The most common way to get them is by IV injection.

2. Angiotensin Converting Enzyme Inhibitors

ACE inhibitors function by preventing the production of a hormone that constricts blood arteries.

3. Calcium Channel Blockers

CCBs function by preventing calcium from entering the cardiac muscles and blood vessels. The blood vessels can now relax as a result.

4. Central Agonists

Central agonists delay nerve impulses, which relaxes blood arteries.

5. Vasodilators

Vasodilators dilate blood arteries to provide proper and swift blood flow.

6. Inhibitors of Renin

Renin-inhibitors reduce the body's natural production of substances that constrict blood vessels and raise blood pressure.

Regrettably, there are several adverse effects associated with high blood pressure drugs. To have a better idea, look below:

1. Breathing difficulties and symptoms of asthma—as a result of using beta-blockers for high blood pressure.

2. Depression—as a result of using beta-blockers for high blood pressure.

3. Issues with having sex—as a result of using beta-blockers for high blood pressure.

4. Hacking cough—an outcome of enzyme inhibitors that convert angiotensin.

5. Skin rash—an outcome of enzyme inhibitors that convert angiotensin.

6. Constipation—because of the calcium channel blockers.

7. Heart palpitations—because of the calcium channel blockers.

8. Frequent headaches—because of the calcium channel blockers.

9. Anemia—the outcome of the Central Agonists.

10. Fever—the outcome of the Central Agonists.

11. Fluid retention —because of the vasodilators.

12. Excessive hair growth—because of the vasodilators.

13. Diarrhea—because of inhibitors of renin.

To reduce blood pressure, it is important to explore other, more effective forms of treatment. Recall that there are several ways in which lifestyle choices can raise blood pressure. Because of this, even little changes to your lifestyle can automatically lower your blood pressure and keep you away from drugs that have negative side effects. The secret is to combine natural therapies with a few lifestyle adjustments.

Consider making the following natural lifestyle changes to achieve normal blood pressure in the future:

1. Frequent Exercise

It should be noted that five days a week, thirty to sixty minutes of moderate exercise can lower blood pressure readings by four to nine millimeters of mercury. In addition, a rigorous exercise regimen can move you out of the danger zone by lowering blood pressure in a matter of weeks.

Exercise also helps to control prehypertension. Recall that systolic pressure over 130 and below 139 or diastolic pressure above 80 and below 89 are indicative of prehypertension.

Consultation with a physician is necessary before starting an exercise regimen. Certain individuals with hypertension must begin at a different dosage. For instance, to start on the path to recovery, some sedentary persons should only exercise for ten minutes each day.

Keep in mind that exercising exclusively on the weekends—a strategy that many individuals with hectic schedules use—does more damage than good. Elevating the physical activity level to a drastic degree might aggravate heart obstruction. Never forget that your heart needs time to acclimate to physical exertion.

2. Lose Weight While Keeping the Scale Number in Check

The number on the scale naturally corresponds to high blood pressure. Even a ten-pound weight loss can lower blood pressure and make any blood pressure drugs that are currently in use more effective.

Keep in mind that not every weight is made equal. It's critical to avoid carrying excess weight around the waist. Take a look at the following data to see why:

A. woman's risk of developing high blood pressure increases if her waist circumference is 35 inches or more.

B. Men who have a waist circumference of 40 inches or more are more prone to develop high blood pressure.

C. Asian women who have a waist circumference of 32 inches or more are more prone to experience high blood pressure.

D. Asian males who measure 36 inches or more around the waist are more prone to high blood pressure.

3. Limit Your Sodium Intake

As previously established, salt contributes significantly to high blood pressure. Lowering the amount of salt in the diet can lower blood pressure by as much as eight millimeters of mercury. A person's daily salt consumption should not exceed 2,300 mg. African Americans and those over fifty who are more likely to have high blood pressure should aim to maintain daily totals of around 1,500 mg.

Consider the following advice to limit your intake of sodium:

A. Consistently check food labels and choose products with less salt.

B. Record your daily sodium intake in a food journal.

C. Avoid seasoning meals with salt. Exactly 2,300 mg of sodium is included in one teaspoon of salt, which is your daily allowance. Use spices or herbs instead of just adding salt.

D. Steer clear of the freezer area, which is filled with a lot of foods high in salt and preservatives; also, stay away from processed meats, bacon, and potato chips.

E. Cut back on salt consumption day by day. Reduce your sodium intake one day at a time if you have a salt craving so you can get used to the taste.

4. Learn to Eat Well

Maintaining normal values and lowering blood pressure requires eating a colorful, healthful diet. Focus on foods that are low in fat, saturated fat, and cholesterol, such as fruits, vegetables, and whole grains. This has the most significant effect of all, lowering blood pressure readings by 14 mmHg.

Dietary Approaches to Stop Hypertension, or DASH diet, is a blood pressure-healthy eating regimen.

A. Increase potassium levels.

As previously established, potassium helps your body's cells maintain a general sodium equilibrium. Look to fruits and vegetables instead of vitamins in tablet form.

B. Jot down every meal you eat.

Make sure to keep track of everything you consume by recording all of your food in a little diary. In this manner, you may become more aware of your behaviors and adjust them as needed in the future.

C. Make a list before you go to the grocery shop.

Without a plan, you frequently leave the grocery store with junk food and harmful snacks. Steer clear of junk food and use your meal list to focus on your nutritional objectives. It's crucial to keep reading food labels as you make your way around the grocery shop.

D. Treat yourself (sometimes).

Recall that the DASH diet involves a lifestyle change. That doesn't imply, though, that you have to give up on your favorite foods forever. Keep in mind that moderation is the key to everything, and your blood pressure won't suffer much if you sometimes crave a candy bar.

For more information on the DASH Diet, see a later chapter. You may also discover many recipes to help you get started on the path to recovery.

5. Reduce alcohol consumption.

Recall that a relatively modest amount of alcohol may cause a four mmHg drop in blood pressure. But after a couple more drinks, that first shield disappears without a trace. Men should limit their alcohol consumption to two drinks per day, while women should limit their intake to one. Blood pressure levels can rise significantly by consuming too much alcohol (many mmHg). Moreover, it may lessen the overall efficacy of the drugs now prescribed for high blood pressure.

Take a look at these suggestions to cut back on alcohol intake:

A. Record your alcohol consumption.

Maintaining an alcohol journal is crucial, just like keeping a diet or salt diary. Recall that one drink consists of twelve ounces of beer, five ounces of wine, and one and a half ounces of liquor. Keep note of your daily alcohol consumption to monitor your present lifestyle choices.

B. Reduce your drinking one day at a time.

Change the amount of alcohol you consume by cutting back one day at a time, like a taper. If you typically have three drinks, limit yourself to just two today. Gradually continue your transition to less alcohol.

C. Get rid of excessive drinking habits

When you have more than four drinks in one sitting, your blood pressure spikes, which can lead to several unfavorable health issues.

6. Reduce Stress with Meditation and Mindfulness

Anxiety and stress can cause sudden increases in blood pressure, which over time can become chronic. To relieve yourself of your worries, try the mindfulness meditation that follows. Recognize the source of your tension and disengage from your anxious thoughts.

Transcendental meditation is one of the age-old methods being studied by researchers at the College of Maharishi Vedic Medicine in Fairfield, Iowa, to naturally decrease blood pressure. The chief physician, Robert Schneider, MD, claims that transcendental meditation helps practitioners achieve a state of peaceful alertness and awareness of their larger body. Transcendental meditation has been shown to reduce stress by bringing about biochemical changes that enhance the body's innate healing abilities. It is critical to control stress because it is one of the main causes of high blood pressure.

In transcendental meditation, practitioners are advised to select a word or phrase—often called a mantra—that they may repeat repeatedly to induce a state of relaxation. To support this internal self-healing, people are supposed to spend around twenty minutes, twice a day, sitting comfortably with their eyes closed and repeating that mantra.

About 189 out of 213 participants in a recent transcendental meditation research had indicators of lowered blood pressure after practicing transcendental meditation for more than three weeks.

Thus, locate a peaceful, quiet, and dark area for oneself. Say a word or phrase to yourself—for example, "peace"—again and over for around twenty minutes. Repetition of these words will provide your brain with a much-needed respite from the tensions of the present. It can concentrate on fortification and restoration.

7. Give Up Smoking and Avoid Exposure to Secondhand Smoke

In the hour following the last cigarette, nicotine can raise blood pressure by more than 10 mmHg. This implies that those who smoke continuously throughout the day raise their blood pressure, which causes stress to constantly exist between the arteries and blood flow.

In addition, breathing in secondhand cigarette smoke raises the risk of high blood pressure and heart disease.

8. Limit Your Coffee Consumption

Blood pressure can automatically jump while drinking caffeinated beverages like soda and coffee, but it's presently unclear if these spikes are long-lasting or just transient.

It's critical to comprehend how caffeine affects your body specifically. Use an at-home blood pressure monitor to check your blood pressure thirty minutes after consuming your next cup of coffee. Your blood pressure is susceptible to the effects of coffee, so if your readings are higher by ten mmHG, you should cut back on your intake.

The Significance of Blood Pressure Monitoring at Home

Following a diagnosis of hypertension, it's critical to continuously check blood pressure readings every day. While at-home monitoring can provide the doctor with a more accurate picture of the real pressure in the arteries, the doctor's office can only begin a kind of one-moment snapshot. Moreover, a variety of factors, including emotions, present dietary habits, and any drugs taken, might cause changes in blood pressure. The guesswork is eliminated with at-home monitoring.

However, it's crucial to comprehend the distinction between left- and right-arm blood pressure before starting at-home blood pressure monitoring. Typically, there should be no more than a 10 mmHg differential between the two arms. Additionally, one should always test the upper arm for at-home readings rather than the lower arm if one arm typically has greater blood pressure than the other.

Take a look at these guidelines for easy blood pressure monitoring at home:

1. Verify that the blood pressure cuff fits properly at all times. The monitor must properly fit around your upper arm.

2. Aim to avoid caffeine or soda consumption, exercise, and cigarette smoking for thirty minutes before at-home assessments.

3. Acquire the skill of sitting while reading. Always sit in a solid hard-backed chair made of plastic or wood, with your back supported and your head upright. Lay your arms on a table with your upper arms parallel to your heart, and rest your feet flat on the floor. The center of your internal elbow should be above the middle of your cuff.

4. Consistently take three readings, separated by one minute.

5. Make a note of each reading you do, being sure to include the date and time of the reading. Make sure you provide your readings to your physician.

6. Recall that an ideal blood pressure reading is around 120/80 mmHg. Verify whether your blood pressure is normal, prehypertensive, or in stages 1 or 2 of high.

7. You should get medical attention right away if your diastolic or systolic numbers are greater than 110 or 180, respectively.

Various Types of At-Home Blood Pressure Monitors

Keep in mind that there are three essential components to any blood pressure monitor, which you should seek when shopping for an at-home model: an inflated cuff, a read-out gauge, and sometimes a stethoscope. These at-home monitors are available at many pharmacies and medical supply stores.

A. Cuff:

The rubber cuff of the at-home monitor has a nylon fastening. The cuff will pinch your arm and fill with air while you take your blood pressure.

B. Gauge:

Keep in mind that most at-home monitors are digital or aneroid. An arrow on the gauge dial of an aneroid monitor points to the figures representing your blood pressure.

C. Stethoscope:

A stethoscope, which is used to listen to the blood flow from the brachial artery to the elbow, is occasionally included with blood pressure monitors. But these noises are really hard to grasp if you're not trained to hear them. The data from this sound may be recorded for you by modern digital blood pressure monitors.

CHAPTER 6:

SAIT MYTHS EXPOSED: UNDERSTANDING THE TRUTH BEHIND WHAT'S IN THE TABLE SHAKER

Numerous factors can lead to high blood pressure. Reducing salt consumption is, of course, one of the most often recommended strategies to decrease blood pressure levels. As previously noted, the recommended daily consumption of salt is just 2,300 mg, and those who are more susceptible to high blood pressure should only take 1,500 mg.

However, examining the history of salt raises several other issues. Of course, salt is something that people should avoid eating. But what if we realized that the type of salt that enters our bodies through our diet matters when it comes to blood pressure levels?

All minerals, mineral supplements, and electrolytes are essentially salt forms with a small amount of vitamin C added. By simply salting their greens, the Romans created "salad" some thousand years ago. Due to their constant movement, which demanded a quick salt intake, Roman troops were compensated with salt sacks. To survive, their bodies needed salt to control the process of detoxification.

So, why do people demonize salt?

Regrettably, salt has evolved into a type of junk food in our day and age. It's referred to as table salt and doesn't provide any of the minerals and health advantages of its bygone heyday when it was sea salt. The Cambrian layer, which is a layer beneath the ground that is rich in iron, minerals, and a host of other things your body needs to survive and function properly, is where sea salt is generated.

Factories use sea salt and boil it till it turns into table salt. The trace minerals that are extracted from sea salt are cooked and then sold to chemical firms. These firms are effectively taking these nutrients from you, which your body needs to survive.

Table salt, or sodium chloride, is what the businesses offer you as leftover "salt." And everything from potato chips to frozen dinners, Fruit Loops to pasta is preserved with sodium chloride. After consuming these foods for their whole lives, people discover they have high blood pressure and are 65 years old.

Naturally, keep in mind that sea salt has the same amount of sodium as ordinary table salt. But with those extra minerals added, like potassium and manganese, your body can mend itself, regulate itself, and function toward improved overall health.

Additionally, keep in mind that your body needs a steady balance of potassium and salt—yes, salt—to function and cleanse itself. Your body is less prone to build those plaque layers along the artery walls if you detoxify more thoroughly. Blood crystals have a lower chance of causing high blood pressure to develop.

As a result, while considering the "salt scare," keep in mind that you should increase your potassium intake and use sea salt sparingly. You can control your blood pressure with this equilibrium. Because table salt is poisonous, throw it in the garbage. Because table salt is only sodium chloride in its most basic form and has been completely depleted of all nutrients and minerals, it raises blood pressure in the body.

CHAPTER 7:

LOWER BLOOD PRESSURE WITH DIET ALTERATIONS: SUPERFOODS, COOKING OILS, AND ESSENTIAL HERBS

To reduce blood pressure without using medicine, look to a ready-made, colorful food plan. You may naturally minimize the risk of significant health conditions and blood pressure by learning how to use oils, superfoods, and key minerals.

Understanding Dietary Changes to Lower Blood Pressure

1. Increase Calcium, Magnesium, and Potassium Intake

Recall that we discussed the numerous health benefits of sea salt's minerals in the previous chapter. Even though traditional blood pressure knowledge justifies a decrease in sodium, research indicates that consuming foods high in macrominerals, such as sea salt, is considerably more crucial than always avoiding sodium. Recall that humans must maintain a proper ratio of potassium to sodium, therefore increasing current potassium consumption is significantly more crucial than concentrating on low sodium.

It's crucial to include the following in your diet to increase your intake of potassium:

(a) Baked potato with skin for 1081 mg of potassium.

(b) 1 cup Plantains for 716 mg of potassium.

(c) ½ Halibut filet for 840 mg of potassium.

(d) 1 cup of parsnips for 573 mg of potassium.

(e) Sweet potato with skin (694 mg potassium).

Beet greens, roasted duck, pumpkin, mushrooms, tomatoes, and bananas are some other delectable foods that are high in potassium.

Recall that the goal of consuming around 4,700 mg of potassium daily is to naturally reduce blood pressure. Moreover, do not advocate for low-carbohydrate diets in any aspect of your life. Ultimately, white and sweet potatoes are rich in magnesium and potassium.

In addition, dairy products, almonds, fish with bones, bone broth, and leafy greens all contain calcium. Aim for 600 mg of calcium every day to help reduce blood pressure.

2. Reduced Consumption of Carbohydrates, Particularly from Sugars and Refined Carbohydrates

Recall that elevated blood pressure is a result of both insulin resistance and high blood sugar. Moreover, those with high blood pressure are typically found to have chronically high blood sugar and high triglycerides.

All of the foregoing problems are brought on by a high intake of refined grains, processed sugars, and a lot of carbs, which should be regularly checked.

Many argue that consuming fructose raises blood pressure, however further study shows that fructose is not the cause of the issue and that eating fruit and honey, which naturally include fructose, may improve one's health and wellbeing.

3. For calcium and vitamin K2, go to grass-fed ghee, butter, and cheese.

Dairy products from grass-fed cows are loaded with calcium and vitamin K2, both of which can significantly lower blood pressure. Vitamin K2 is a necessary vitamin that shouldn't be excluded from the diet since it offers further protection against osteoporosis, cardiovascular disease, and cancer.

Additionally, vitamin K2 helps to lessen artery calcification and vascular hardness. Moreover, elevated calcium levels contribute to the deposition of calcium in the bones as opposed to the arteries, hence elevating hypertension.

Supplemental vitamin K2 is recommended for those with dairy allergies. To get optimum health, look for pills that include the minerals K2, D, and A.

4. Tea Drinking to Reduce Blood Pressure

Tea drinkers frequently have reduced blood pressure. Recall that certain teas are better than others at lowering blood pressure and that teas with caffeine raise blood pressure initially. To help you decide where to begin your healing process, consider the following teas:

A. Hawthorn tea

A plant included in hawthorn tea has been used to treat heart problems for about two millennia. It dilates blood vessels, facilitates better blood flow, and is high in antioxidants.

B. Hibiscus tea

Because it contains a high concentration of minerals, flavonoids, and other vital elements, hibiscus tea lowers blood pressure. About three cups a day are advised by experts to reap the necessary advantages.

C. Gotu Kola tea

Kola tea is essential for preserving the health of internal connective tissues, which enhances circulation and fortifies veins that are already weak. This prevents plaque fractures, which might result in blood clots.

5. Fatty fish for Omega 3s

Omega-3 fatty acids, which are critical for enhancing cardiovascular health, are abundant in fatty fish. Supplements containing fish oil may also help lower blood pressure on both the systolic and diastolic levels.

It's crucial to eat fatty fish, such as salmon and/or halibut, as they have been shown to contain potassium, which is necessary for a diet that promotes heart health. You can significantly lower your risk of high blood pressure and cardiovascular disease by eating one pound of "fatty" fish every week.

Reduce Blood Pressure with Nutritious Superfoods

Superfoods are great sources of essential nutrients that the body can quickly incorporate into its structure to produce greater, more vibrant health. These nutrients include vitamins, minerals, and antioxidants. For the next few weeks, consuming the following meals can help you feel more energy and lower your overall systolic and diastolic values.

1. Skim Milk

Calcium and vitamin D, which are abundant in skim milk, can help reduce blood pressure by up to ten percent overall. Keep in mind that skim milk, at 382 mg per serving, is much more potassium-rich.

Additionally, skim milk helps to lessen fat and cholesterol blockages, which raise blood pressure because, well, you know.

2. Avocadoes

Potassium, which is abundant in avocados, helps lower blood pressure and is necessary for a general body cleanse. Avocados are also a great source of vitamins, phytonutrients, and monounsaturated fats.

3. Spinach

Because spinach has a high folate content, it helps lower blood pressure. Additionally, spinach is a rich source of proteins, potassium, and magnesium—minerals that help to control the levels of salt crystals in the blood and detoxify the body. Keep in mind that blockages might result from salt crystals building up in the blood.

4. Garlic

Garlic removes fat deposits from the arteries, preventing blockages and coronary heart disease. Garlic also produces gas in the stomach and intestines, which lowers blood pressure and relaxes arterial pressure.

5. Beans

Rich in protein, fiber, iron, potassium, magnesium, and other vital elements, beans are incredibly nutritious. Moreover, a cup of beans has around 12 grams of fiber or half of what women should consume daily. Because they are high in fiber and make you feel full and satisfied for extended periods, research suggests that beans may help you lose weight.

6. Almonds

Nutrients included in almonds, including good fats, vitamins, and minerals, can decrease blood pressure and total cholesterol. Frequent almond eating can raise HDL, the "good cholesterol," and lower LDL, the "bad cholesterol." Almonds also combat diabetes and cardiovascular illnesses, two conditions that raise blood pressure.

Making the Cooking Oil Switch

Take note that cutting back on salt and saturated fat intake is advised by the American Heart Association. Margarine and butter should thus be avoided. Replace your current cooking oils with these to reduce blood pressure and revitalize your nutritious cooking.

1. Safflower Oil

The spiny plate is used to make safflower oil, which has just 9% saturated fat, 13% monounsaturated fat, and 78% polyunsaturated fat. It's great when cooked veggies or sprinkled over salads.

2. Canola Oil

The rapeseed plant is used to make canola oil, which has a high content of polyunsaturated fats and just 7% saturated fats.

3. Soybean Oil

Soybean oil has a stunning 61 percent polyunsaturated fat and only 13 percent saturated fat.

4, Sunflower Oil

Vitamin E, which is abundant in sunflower oil, aids in restoring blood pressure to normal. The majority of people ought to take at least 15 mg daily.

5. Olive Oil

Good monounsaturated fats, such as those found in olive oil, help to decrease blood pressure and reduce the risk of heart disease.

Herbal Remedies for Blood Pressure

See how you may use the following herbs and supplements to add excellent taste and reduce blood pressure in your regular cooking. The following herbs are particularly good at bringing down blood pressure:

1. Cinnamon

Try using cinnamon, particularly if you have diabetes, to lower your blood pressure. Use this flavor-boosting spice for a boost of flavor in your coffee, cereal, or oatmeal.

2. Basil

Basil is a simple plant to grow in your yard and, when consumed, immediately decreases blood pressure, providing your arteries with much-needed respite.

3. Garlic

Your blood vessels will relax as a result of eating garlic, improving blood flow and cellular oxygenation.

4. Cardamom

An Indian plant called cardamom is known to reduce blood pressure. It adds an interesting taste to stews, soups, and meat rubs.

5. Celery Seed

Ancient Chinese medicine employed celery, which has been demonstrated to be effective in treating hypertension.

6. Cat's Claw

Cat's claw reduces the severity of your hypertension and replenishes the calcium channels in your body.

CHAPTER 8:

20-DASH DIET RECIPES: APPETIZERS, MAIN DISHES, AND DESSERTS

Heart Healthy

Appetizer Recipes

Ginger and Balsamic Marinated Mushrooms

Yield: 4 Per Servings

Nutrition information Per Serving:

Calories: 65 calories

Sodium: 15 mg

Carbohydrates: 13 g

Fat: 1g

Protein: 3 g

Ingredients:

- 4 Portobello mushrooms

- 3/4 cup pineapple juice

- 1/3 cup balsamic vinegar

- 2 ½ tbsp. chopped and peeled ginger

- 1 tbsp. chopped basil

Directions:

First, put the cleaned and de-stemmed mushrooms, their gill-like side facing up, in a small glass dish.

Next, in a separate dish, combine the vinegar, ginger, and pineapple juice. Cover the glass dish with the marinated mushrooms and refrigerate for one hour to enable the marinade to work its magic.

Next, get a charcoal grill ready or preheat a gas grill. Before serving, grill the mushrooms for five minutes on each side and top with basil. Have fun!

Rosemary Potato Skins

Yield: 2 Per Servings

Nutrition information Per Serving:

Calories: 114

Sodium: 18 g.

Carbohydrates: 27 g

Fat: 0 g

Protein: 2 g

Ingredients:

- 2 medium-sized potatoes

- 1½ tbsp finely chopped rosemary

- 1/4 teaspoons of black pepper

- olive oil

Directions:

Preheat the oven to 375 degrees Fahrenheit.

After cleaning, pierce the potatoes with a fork to make holes in them. After placing the potatoes on a baking pan, bake them for an hour.

Next, cut the potatoes in half and scoop out the insides, leaving about an eighth inch of the insides still connected to the skin. The insides of the potato can be saved for another occasion.

Lightly brush each potato skin with a little olive oil, then evenly distribute the pepper and rosemary. Re-enter the oven and cook the skins for 10 minutes. Enjoy them right away after serving.

Paprika and Lemon Hummus

Yield: 14 Pre Servings

Nutritional Information Per Serving:

Calories: 80

Sodium: 180 mg

Carbohydrates: 10 g

Fat: 3 g

Protein: 3 g

Ingredients:

- 32 ounces of low-sodium canned chickpeas

- 3 minced garlic cloves

- 1 tablespoon olive oil

- ⅓ cup lemon juice

- ½ teaspoon paprika

- ¼ teaspoons of black pepper

- 2 tbsp. sesame paste

- 2 ½ tsp finely chopped parsley

Directions:

Transfer the chickpeas to a food processor, being careful not to add any of the canning liquid. Once the chickpeas are pureed, add the tahini, olive oil, parsley, garlic, lemon juice, pepper, and paprika. Keep puréeing the liquid. The liquid from the can of chickpeas should then be added to the processor gradually until the appropriate consistency is reached. Have fun.

Delicious Dijon Mustard-Based Shrimp

Yield: 8 Per Servings

Nutritional Information Per Serving:

Calories: 70

Sodium: 200 mg

Carbohydrates: 3 g

Fat: 1 g

Protein: 12 g

Ingredients:

- 1 pound peeled and deveined raw shrimp

- 1 onion (diced)

- ⅓ cup lime juice

- 3 tbsp Dijon mustard

- 1 tbsp capers

- 1 cup of water

- ⅓ cup rice vinegar

- 1 bay leaf.

- 3 cloves

Directions:

Mix the mustard, onion, capers, and lime juice first. Place the ingredients in a small baking dish, stir well, and put aside.

Then, combine the cloves, vinegar, water, and bay leaf in a skillet or saucepan. Let the mixture come to a boil. Add the shrimp to the mixture after they start to boil. Stir them constantly and let them cook for a full minute. Once the mixture has been drained, add the shrimp to the baking dish with onions. Be careful to discard the bay leaf and cloves first. Before serving, give the mixture in the baking dish a good stir and let it cool in the fridge for an hour.

Superfood Sunday Dip with Avocado

Yield: 4 Per Servings

Nutrition Information Per Serving:

Calories: 80

Sodium: 50 mg

Carbohydrates: 8 g

Fat: 5 g

2 g of protein

Ingredients:

- 1 peeled and mashed avocado

- ½ cup sour cream

- ¼ teaspoon hot sauce

- 3 tsp chopped onion

Directions:

Add the avocado, chopped onion, sour cream, and spicy sauce and stir until well blended. Enjoy the dip with some veggies on the side!

Heart Healthy

Main Courses

Mediterranean Chicken Salad

Yield: 4 Per Servings

Nutrition Information Per Serving:

Calories: 250

Sodium: 264 mg

Carbohydrates: 14 g

Fat: 7 g.

Protein: 29 g

Ingredients:

- 4 boneless, skinless chicken breasts

- 3 minced garlic cloves

- 6 cups of lettuce greens

- 1 cup of black olives

- 2 sliced oranges

Salad Dressing Ingredients:

- ½ Cup red wine vinegar

- 1 tablespoon olive oil

- 5 garlic cloves minced

- 1 tbsp diced onion

- 1 tbsp. chopped celery

- 1 tsp. black pepper

Directions:

First, make the dressing. Mix the olive oil, celery, garlic, vinegar, onion, and pepper. Refrigerate the mixture by covering it.

After that, coat the chicken breasts with garlic and cook them in a pan for five minutes on each side. As soon as possible, put the chicken on a chopping board and let it cool. Then cut it into the proper number of strips.

Divide the chicken, lettuce, oranges, and olives into four halves. Top each salad with a dollop of the prepared dressing. Have fun.

Chicken Paella

Yield: 4 Per Servings

Nutrition Information Per Serving:

Calories: 375

Sodium: 180 mg

Carbohydrates: 45 g

Fat: 6 g

Protein: 35 g

Ingredients:

- 1 pound chicken breasts, skinless and boneless

- 1 teaspoon olive oil

- 1 onion, chopped

- 3 leeks, sliced

- 4 minced garlic cloves

- 2 tomatoes, diced

- 1 cup of brown rice

- 1 pepper, sliced

- 1 teaspoon tarragon

- 1 cup of peas

- 2 cups chicken broth

- 1 lemon sliced

- ⅓ cup parsley

Directions:

In a frying pan, warm the olive oil over medium heat to start. Add the chicken, leeks, garlic, and onions to the frying pan and simmer for five minutes. Add the tomatoes and peppers after that, and simmer the mixture for a further five minutes.

Lastly, include the rice, stock, and tarragon into the mixture and heat it all to a boil.

Turn the heat down to medium-low and cover the pot after it starts to boil. Before adding the peas, let the stew boil for 10 minutes. Give the mixture a full hour to boil.

Present the paella and savor it!

Asian-Inspired Pork Tenderloin

Yield: 2 Per Servings

Nutrition Information Per Serving:

Calories: 246

Sodium: 55 mg

Carbohydrates: 0 g

Fat: 16 g

Protein: 26

Ingredients:

- 1/2 pound sliced pork tenderloin

- 1 tbsp sesame seeds

- ⅛ teaspoon cayenne pepper

- ⅛ teaspoon celery seed

- ½ teaspoon coriander

- ⅛ teaspoon cinnamon

- ⅛ teaspoon cumin

- 1 tablespoon sesame oil

Directions:

Preheat the oven to 400 degrees Fahrenheit.

Then, arrange the sesame seeds in a frying pan in a single layer. Make sure the seeds brown after cooking them for around two minutes.

Combine the onion, coriander, cumin, cayenne, cinnamon, toasted sesame seeds, and sesame oil in a separate bowl.

After putting the tenderloin in a baking dish, coat it with the spices, being careful to coat all sides equally. Place the pork in the prepared oven and bake for fifteen minutes, then serve.

Hungry Man Beef Stew

Yield: 4 Per Servings

Nutrition Information Per Serving:

Calories: 380

Sodium: 165 mg

Carbohydrates: 35 g

Fat: 9 g

Protein: 42 g

Ingredients:

- 1 pound beef

- 1 cup of celery, chopped

- 2 diced onions

- 1 cup of tomatoes, diced

- 2 tsp olive oil

- ⅓ cup chopped sweet potato

- ½ cup chopped mushrooms

- ½ cup chopped potato

- 4 garlic cloves, minced

- 1 cup kale (diced)

- ⅓ cup red wine vinegar

- ⅓ cup of barley

- 2 tsp of balsamic vinegar

- 1 tsp of crushed sage

- 3 cups of vegetable broth.

- 1-tablespoon oregano

- 1-tablespoon parsley

- 1 teaspoon rosemary

Directions:

Cut the meat and veggies into thin slices and dice first. In a slow cooker, combine all the ingredients and stir. After that, simmer the stew for 10 hours on LOW.

Warm and enjoy!

Grilled Halibut with Homemade Salsa

Yield: 4 Per Servings

Nutrition Information Per Serving:

Calories: 125

Sodium: 80 mg

Carbohydrates: 3 g

Fat: 4g

Protein: 22 g

Ingredients:

- 4-ounce halibut filets

- 2 tomatoes, diced

- 1 teaspoon chopped oregano

- 2 ½ tbsp. chopped basil

- 3 tsp. olive oil

- 2 minced garlic cloves

Directions:

Preheat the oven to 350 degrees Fahrenheit.

Add the tomato, garlic, oregano, and basil after that. Stir the mixture after adding the olive oil until it is all incorporated.

Arrange the halibut filets on a baking sheet, then cover the fish with the tomato mixture. After fifteen minutes of cooking, serve the filets.

Maple-Glazed Salmon

Yield: 6 Per Servings

Nutrition Information Per Serving:

Calories: 250

Sodium: 150 mg

Carbohydrates: 10 g

Fat: 10 g

Protein: 30 g

Ingredients:

- 2 pounds of salmon sliced

- ⅓ cup maple syrup

- 2 minced garlic cloves

- ⅓ cup balsamic vinegar

- ½ teaspoon sea salt

- ¼ tsp of black pepper

Directions:

Preheat the oven to 450 degrees Fahrenheit.

Then, combine the maple syrup, garlic, and balsamic vinegar; warm the mixture over low heat. Pour half of this mixture into a bowl and save the other half for a later stage after cooking for approximately five minutes.

Arrange the salmon on a baking sheet and coat it with the mixture that was made.
Oven-bake the fish for ten minutes. Then apply the mixture to the fish once more. Five more minutes of baking are needed. After that, take out the salmon once again and baste. For the following twenty-five minutes, keep doing this.

Enjoy the fish later with a dollop of the maple syrup you saved.

Sea Scallops with Lime

Yield: 4 Per Servings

Nutrition Information Per Serving:

Calories: 200

Sodium: 184 mg

22 g carbohydrate

Fat: 4g

Protein: 19 g

Ingredients:

- 1 pound of sea scallops

- 5 tbsp honey

- 1 tablespoon olive oil

- 3 tablespoons lime juice

- 3-tsp grated lime peel

- 1 lime, sliced

Directions:

Heat your broiler first. Line a broiler pan with aluminum foil, end to end.

Combine the honey, oil, and lime juice in a separate bowl. After applying this mixture to the scallops, put them on the broiler pan. Scallions should be broiled for five minutes. Then turn the scallions over and cook for another minute.

Transfer the scallions to heated plates and drizzle with more lemon juice for extra flavor. Enjoy after adding the lime slices and peel on top.

Asparagus and Goat Cheese Penne Pasta

Yield: 2 Per Servings

Nutrition Information Per Serving:

Calories: 390

Sodium: 140 mg

Carbohydrates: 64 g

Fat: 8 g

Protein: 17 g

Ingredients:

- ½ cup of cherry tomatoes, sliced

- ½ cup chopped asparagus

- 2 tbsp water

- ⅓ pound whole wheat pasta (I used penne)

- ⅓ cup finely chopped basil

- ¼ teaspoon black pepper

- 2 garlic cloves, minced

- 3 ounces goat cheese

Directions:

Start by adding more water to a large saucepan until it is halfway full and letting it boil. Once it starts to boil, add the pasta to the water and cook until it becomes soft. Once it's done, take out the pasta.

Transfer the asparagus to a bowl with a tablespoon of water, then microwave on high for three minutes.

Combine the pasta, asparagus, goat cheese, garlic, basil, tomatoes, and pepper on the side. Until the creation is fully integrated, discard it. Before

serving, let the pasta chill in the refrigerator for 30 minutes.
Enjoy.

Vegetable Quinoa Risotto

Yield: 6 Per Servings

Nutrition Information Per Serving:

Calories: 150

Sodium: 290 mg

Carbohydrates: 23 g

Fat: 3 g

Protein: 8 g

Ingredients:

- 1 onion, chopped

- 2 minced garlic cloves

- 1 tablespoon olive oil

- 1 cup of quinoa

- 2 cups arugula, diced

- 2 ½ cups vegetable stock

- ⅓ cup Parmesan cheese

- ½ cup mushrooms, sliced

- ¼ teaspoon salt

- ¼ teaspoon pepper

Directions:

In a pot, first heat the olive oil, onion, and garlic. Let the onion get transparent. The quinoa should then be added and cooked for one minute.

After that, add the stock to the pot and bring it to a boil. After putting the mixture on low heat, let it simmer for twelve minutes. The mixture will then be foamy.

When the quinoa is transparent, add the mushrooms
and arugula and cook the mixture further.

Stir in the cheese, salt, and pepper. Warm up and
serve.

Thyme for Basil Pizza

Yield: 4 Per Servings

Nutrition Information Per Serving:

Calories: 175

Sodium: 275 mg

Carbohydrates: 32 g

Fat: 2 g

Protein: 8 g

Ingredients:

- 12-inch pizza crust (from the grocery store)

- ½ cup no-fat ricotta cheese

- 5 minced garlic cloves

- ⅓ cup sun-dried tomatoes

- 1 teaspoon thyme

- 2 tsp basil

Directions:

Preheat the oven to 425 degrees Fahrenheit.

After that, put the pizza crust on a pan and cover it with the cheese, tomatoes, and garlic. After straining the thyme and basil over the ingredients, bake the pizza for 20 minutes. Serve warm.

Heart Healthy

Desserts

Spiced Carrot Bread

Yield: 17 Per Servings

Nutrition Information Per Serving:

Calories: 100

Sodium: 130 mg

Carbohydrates: 15 g

Fat: 4g

Protein: 2 g

Ingredients:

- 1 cup of whole wheat flour

- ⅓ cup all-purpose flour

- ½ teaspoon baking soda

- 2 tsp of baking powder

- 1 tsp cinnamon

- ½ teaspoon ginger

- ⅓ cup brown sugar

- ⅓ cup no trans fat buttery blend

- ⅓ cup of skim milk

- 2 egg white alternatives

- 2 tbsp orange juice, no sugar added

- 1 ½ teaspoon grated orange rind

- 1 teaspoon vanilla

- 1 ⅓ cup carrots, shredded

- 1 tablespoon chopped walnuts

- 3 tsp of golden raisins

Directions:

Preheat the oven to 375 degrees Fahrenheit.

In a small bowl, start by combining the flour, baking powder, baking soda, cinnamon, and ginger. Place this dish aside.

Combine the brown sugar, buttery blend, skim milk, egg white replacements, orange juice, vanilla, and orange rind in a separate, bigger bowl. Next, gradually add the walnuts, carrots, and raisins while stirring constantly. Finally, stir in the remaining flour mixture. Mix thoroughly.

After that, transfer the batter to a bread pan and bake it for 45 minutes. Before serving, let the bread cool for five minutes.

Enjoy.

Hazel Pumpkin Afternoon Cake

Yield: 12 Per Servings

Nutrition Information Per Serving:

Calories: 175

Sodium: 80 mg

Carbohydrates: 28 g

Fat: 6 g

Protein: 4 g

Ingredients:

- ⅓ cup honey

- 4 tablespoons canola oil

- 1 cup of pumpkin puree

- 4 tablespoons brown sugar

- 1 cup flour, wholemeal

- 2 eggs

- ⅓ cup all-purpose flour

- ½ teaspoon baking powder

- 3 tablespoons of flaxseed

- 1-tsp. cinnamon

- ½ teaspoon allspice

- ½ teaspoon nutmeg

- ½ teaspoon cloves

- ⅛ teaspoon salt

- 3 tablespoons chopped hazelnuts

Directions:

Preheat the oven to 350 degrees Fahrenheit.

Then, whisk together the pureed pumpkin, eggs, honey, brown sugar, and canola oil.
Be sure to fully combine the ingredients.

Combine flour, baking powder, flaxseed, cinnamon, nutmeg, allspice, salt, and cloves in a small bowl. Make sure all of the ingredients are thoroughly combined by mixing this flour mixture into the pumpkin mixture.

After that, transfer this batter to a pan and sprinkle the hazelnuts on top. After the cake has baked for fifty-five minutes, let it cool before cutting it into pieces. Enjoy

Springtime Strawberry Shortcake

Yield: 8 Per Servings

Nutrient Information Per Serving:

Calories: 220

Sodium: 86 mg

Carbohydrates: 37 g

Fat: 5 g

Protein: 7 g

Ingredients:

- 2 cups whole wheat pastry flour

- 2 ¼ cups baking powder

- ⅛ cup all-purpose flour

- 1½ tablespoons sugar

- 1 cup of skim milk

- ¼ cup no-trans fat margarine

- 5 cups sliced strawberries

- 1 cup fat-free yogurt

Directions:

Preheat the oven to 425 degrees Fahrenheit.

Next, combine the sugar, baking powder, and flour. Using your fingers, cut the margarine into the flour mixture until crumbles form. Stir the mixture just until it's well combined, being careful not to overmix. Pour the milk into the mixture.

After that, put the dough on a surface dusted with flour and use your hands to mix it approximately eight times, ensuring the dough is smooth. Roll out the dough to a thickness of 1/4 inch for a rectangular shape. Cut the dough into square pieces and arrange them on a baking tray. Bake the squares for a total of twelve minutes.

After the biscuits cool, arrange them on plates and serve them with yogurt and strawberries.

Zany Zucchini Bread

Yield: 18 Per Servings

Nutrition Information Per Serving:

Calories: 170

Sodium: 103 mg

Carbohydrates: 25 g

Fat: 5 g

Protein: 4 g

Ingredients:

- ⅓ cup canola oil

- 6 white eggs

- ⅓ cup sugar

- ⅔ cup applesauce

- 2 teaspoons of vanilla

- 1 cup all-purpose flour

- 1 ½ cup of whole-wheat flour

- 1 teaspoon of baking soda

- 1 tsp baking powder

- 3 tsp of cinnamon

- 2 ½ cup shredded finely zucchini

- 1 ⅓ cup crushed pineapple

Directions:

Preheat the oven to 350 degrees Fahrenheit.

Next, in a large dish, combine the applesauce, egg whites, sugar, vanilla, and canola oil.

Combine the flour, baking soda, cinnamon, and baking powder in a separate basin.

Blend the wet and dry components. Stirring constantly, add the pineapple and zucchini last. Thick batter is what's needed.

Transfer this mixture to a loaf pan and bake for fifty minutes.

After letting the bread cool, Serve it!

Spiced Poached Pears

Yield: 4 Per Servings

Nutrition Information Per Serving:

Calories: 140

Sodium: 9 mg

Carbohydrates: 33 g

Fat: 1 g

Protein: 1 g

Ingredients:

- 4 pear

- 1 cup orange juice

- ⅓ cup apple juice

- 1 teaspoon nutmeg

- 1 tsp cinnamon

- 3 tbsp. zest from an orange

- ½ cup raspberries

Directions:

Mix the juice, nutmeg, and cinnamon first.

Subsequently, peel every pear and endeavor to extract the core from the fruit's base. After placing each pear in a pan, cover the pears with the juice mixture.

After putting the pan over medium heat, simmer the juice combination for thirty minutes. Make frequent turns with the pears and avoid letting the mixture boil. After that, add raspberries and orange zest to the pears and serve them warm. Have fun.

Conclusion

You may learn everything you need to know about high blood pressure and how it affects the body from The Blood Pressure Solution. One in three persons in the Western world suffers from high blood pressure, which is a major contributing factor to several conditions including heart disease, stroke, heart attack, diabetes, and kidney failure. It needs to end.

Fortunately, you may lower your high blood pressure readings back to normal if you make lifestyle changes, focus on boosting your health with nutrient-dense, colorful meals, and begin to realize the extreme strain you've been placing on your arteries over the previous several years. Without the costly medicine, you may take steps to get your blood pressure back to normal. You may make all of your decisions with improved health in mind and live your life appropriately. These potential health issues don't have to control you. By controlling your blood pressure, you can prevent heart-wrenching, life-altering illnesses down the road. Fight back against the future you now have and forge a new one. began today.